The Amoxicillin Guidebook

A Comprehensive Guide on how to Completely End
Infections like Pneumonia, Respiratory Tract Infections,
Urinary Tract Infections, Otitis Media, Tooth Infections and
Many More Using Antibiotics Pills

Dr. Quinton Vale

The Amoxicillin Guidebook/ Dr. Quinton Vale -- 1st ed.

CONTENTS

PREFACE

The world of antibiotics has always been a subject of fascination and importance in the field of medicine. Ever since Alexander Fleming discovered penicillin in 1928, antibiotics have been crucial in combating bacterial infections, saving countless lives, and improving patient outcomes. Among the many antibiotics available, Amoxicillin holds a prominent position for its efficacy, safety, and broad applicability in treating various infections. This book aims to serve as a comprehensive guide on how to use Amoxicillin antibiotic pills to effectively end different types of bacterial infections.

Infections are a leading cause of mortality and morbidity globally. The ability to combat them is an essential part of modern healthcare. However, the reckless use of antibiotics has led to the rise of antibiotic-resistant bacteria, making it more critical than ever to use these lifesaving drugs judiciously. This book is intended for both healthcare professionals who prescribe Amoxicillin and for patients who are prescribed this antibiotic. By providing a thorough understanding of Amoxicillin's uses, dosages, potential side effects, and special considerations, this book aims to encourage responsible antibiotic use.

The focus of this guide is not merely to list out the infections that can be treated with Amoxicillin but to offer a holistic understanding. From the mechanism of action to the potential for antibiotic resistance, we cover all aspects that one should be aware of. By arming yourself with this knowledge, you can make informed decisions about your health and play a role in combating the global issue of antibiotic resistance.

This book is divided into several chapters, each dedicated to a different aspect of Amoxicillin and its application in treating infections. It begins by introducing what Amoxicillin is and its mechanism of action. Subsequent chapters discuss the types of infections treatable with this antibiotic, from pneumonia and respiratory tract infections to urinary tract infections and tooth infections. We also delve into dosage and administration guidelines, side effects, drug interactions, and special considerations for specific populations like pregnant women and the elderly. Towards the end of the book, we discuss the pressing issue of antibiotic resistance and how responsible usage can mitigate this problem.

We also include case studies to provide real-world context to the theoretical information. These case studies offer valuable insights into the effectiveness of Amoxicillin in different scenarios, and they also serve as cautionary tales on what can go wrong if the antibiotic is misused.

In the age of information, there is a sea of material available at our fingertips. However, the sheer volume can sometimes lead to misinformation. This book aims to be a reliable resource, substantiated by scientific research and expert opinions. As the saying goes, "Knowledge is power." This book aims to empower its readers with the knowledge needed to use Amoxicillin responsibly and effectively.

Remember, while this book aims to be a comprehensive guide, it is not a substitute for professional medical advice. Always consult with healthcare professionals for diagnosis and treatment of medical conditions.

By the end of this guide, you will have a well-rounded understanding of how Amoxicillin can be used to combat various bacterial infections effectively. Here's to a future where we can continue to rely on antibiotics, like Amoxicillin, to save lives, thanks to responsible use and ongoing scientific research.

INTRODUCTION

Infections, a persistent and ever-evolving challenge to human health, demand our attention and understanding. This chapter marks the beginning of our journey into the intricate world of infections and the pivotal role of Amoxicillin in their resolution.

Infections are the result of harmful microorganisms invading the body and multiplying. These microorganisms can include bacteria, viruses, fungi, and parasites. Infections can affect various parts of the body and have the potential to cause a wide range of health issues.

Understanding infections is crucial for effective treatment and management. In this chapter, we will explore the nature of infections, their causes, the impact they can have on health, and why prompt treatment is essential.

Infections encompass a broad range of diseases and conditions caused by invading microorganisms. They can manifest in various ways and affect different body systems. Common types of infections include bacterial, viral, fungal, and parasitic infections. Each type has its unique characteristics and requires specific approaches to treatment.

To effectively combat infections, we must uncover their sources and routes of transmission. Understanding how infections originate and spread enables us to take proactive measures for prevention and to apply targeted treatments when needed.

Infections can be transmitted through various routes, each presenting distinct challenges and opportunities for prevention. Infections are not mere inconveniences; they possess the power to profoundly influence human health. The consequences of an infection can span from mild, self-limiting symptoms to severe, life-threatening conditions. This section will delve into the diverse impacts of infections on well-being, underscoring the importance of timely intervention and appropriate treatment.

Prompt action in the face of infections is not merely a matter of convenience; it can be a matter of life and death. Untreated or inadequately managed infections can lead to dire consequences for individuals and populations. In this book, we elucidate the critical reasons for the urgency of timely and effective treatment, spotlighting the role of antibiotics, particularly Amoxicillin, in this context.

Swift treatment is instrumental in preventing infections from progressing to more severe stages. Complications such as abscess formation, tissue damage, or the dissemination of infection to vital organs can often be averted with timely medical intervention.

Timely treatment not only benefits the individual but also contributes to reducing the transmission of infections to others. Contagious infections can be curtailed through isolation and appropriate treatment, thereby safeguarding the health of communities.

The judicious use of antibiotics is paramount in preserving their effectiveness.

The importance of antibiotics in the modern world cannot be overstated. The discovery of antibiotics marked a watershed moment in medical history. Before this, simple bacterial infections could escalate into life-threatening conditions, with physicians having little to no effective means to treat them. Antibiotics transformed this grim scenario, offering a reliable way to combat bacterial diseases and drastically reducing mortality rates. In surgeries, childbirth, and the treatment of chronic conditions, antibiotics play a crucial role in preventing bacterial infections, thereby facilitating medical advancements that we often take for granted.

History of Antibiotic Discovery

The discovery of antibiotics in the early 20th century transformed medicine and saved countless lives. However, the road leading to the first antibiotics was long and built on centuries of scientific advances.

Ancient civilizations, including those in Greece, China, and Egypt, unknowingly used antibiotics present in moldy bread or soil to treat infections. However, the organisms responsible were unknown. It was not until the Golden Age of microbiology in the late 1800s that the germ theory of disease took hold, propelling the search for anti-bacterial treatments.

In 1928, Alexander Fleming made the chance discovery of penicillin, the first natural antibiotic, from the Penicillium mold. Fleming observed that colonies of the mold that had contaminated his petri dishes suppressed the growth of staphylococci bacteria. After further tests, he concluded that the mold must secrete a substance capable of killing a variety of disease-causing bacteria.

Fleming published his findings in 1929, noting the potential use of penicillin as an anti-bacterial chemotherapeutic agent. However, Fleming faced difficulties in stabilizing and mass producing the compound. He lacked resources to develop penicillin further despite its promise.

In the 1930s, other researchers, including Howard Florey and Ernst Chain, picked up where Fleming left off. They managed to purify penicillin and conducted trials in mice and humans. By 1941, their team successfully treated systemic infections and published results that garnered wide attention.

With World War II raging, governments poured resources into scaling up production of penicillin. Advances were made in fermentation and purification methods to yield greater supplies. By 1943, penicillin was available in quantity to treat battlefield injuries and infections on the front lines.

The impact of penicillin was immediate and profound. Deaths from bacterial pneumonia, meningitis, gangrene and sepsis plummeted among Allied forces. The Miracle Drug was hailed as a turning point in the war and in modern medicine.

In 1945, Fleming, Florey and Chain were awarded the Nobel Prize in Medicine for the discovery and development of penicillin. By then, penicillin was being mass produced around the world to meet demand. However, microbiologists cautioned early on about the potential for resistance.

Research continued to find new sources of antibiotics in the environment. In 1946, streptomycin was isolated from the actinobacterium Streptomyces griseus, offering an alternative to penicillin. Other soil organisms yielded antibiotics like tetracycline (1948), erythromycin (1952) and vancomycin (1956).

Chemical modification of existing compounds also produced antibiotic derivatives like methicillin (1960s) to overcome resistance. By the 1950s, the "Golden Age" of antibiotics discovery yielded over a hundred compounds, treating a wide spectrum of bacterial infections.

Unfortunately, the rate of new antibiotic discovery slowed by the 1970s. While incremental improvements have been made, no new antibiotic classes have emerged since 1987. With the continued evolution of antibiotic resistance, researchers warn we may enter a "post-antibiotic era" where common infections are untreatable.

The history of antibiotics is a triumph of science and serendipity. But the challenge ahead is developing innovative new treatments before we lose ground against evolving bacteria. Recapturing the collaborative spirit of early antibiotic pioneers will be key.

WHAT IS AMOXICILLIN

Amoxicillin is a semi-synthetic antibiotic that belongs to the penicillin class of antibiotics. It was first developed in the 1970s as an improved version of ampicillin, with better bioavailability when taken orally. Its chemical name is (2S,5R,6R)-6-[(2R)-2-amino-2-(4-hydroxyphenyl)acetyl]amino-3,3-dimethyl-7-oxo-4-thia-1-azabicyclo[3.2.0]heptane-2-carboxylic acid.

The molecular formula for Amoxicillin is $C_{16}H_{19}N_{3}O_{5}S$, and it has a molecular weight of approximately 365.4 grams per mole. Its chemical structure consists of a beta-lactam ring, which is crucial for its antibacterial activity, attached to an amino group. The presence of this amino group enhances its solubility and absorption, making it more effective when administered orally compared to other penicillins.

Development of Amoxicillin

The first-generation penicillins like penicillin G had limitations. They were only effective against Gram-positive bacteria but inactive against the Gram-negative pathogens increasingly causing community infections. Penicillins also faced growing resistance from penicillinase enzymes that degraded the drug.

Pharmaceutical companies wanted to create penicillin derivatives able to withstand penicillinases while treating a broader range of bacteria. The search began for what would be known as aminopenicillins.

In 1962, Beecham Research Laboratories chemists selected an acyl side chain variant of ampicillin for further testing. Ampicillin itself was developed a decade earlier as a broader spectrum penicillin. The new compound, designated Beecham 1652, showed promise resisting penicllinases.

After promising preclinical studies, Beecham launched clinical trials in 1964 comparing their experimental antibiotic against other available therapies. Results confirmed it was highly active against common Gram-positive and Gram-negative pathogens while having low toxicity.

In 1972, Beecham 1652 received approval by the FDA under the brand name Amoxil. It was the second aminopenicillin brought to market after ampicillin. Amoxicillin proved superior in absorption and tolerability compared to earlier penicillins.

Unlike penicillin G, amoxicillin is well-absorbed orally with a bioavailability of 75-92%. It also has a longer serum half-life enabling less frequent dosing. Such pharmacokinetic properties made amoxicillin ideal for outpatient treatment of community infections.

During the 1970s and 1980s, amoxicillin rapidly became a globally prescribed antibiotic for bacterial illness. It remains one of the most commonly prescribed antibiotics today, especially for pediatric patients. Reasons include its broad spectrum coverage, high tissue penetration, and favorable safety profile.

Amoxicillin has activity against both Gram-positive cocci like Streptococcus pneumoniae, the causative bacteria of pneumonia and meningitis, as well as Gram-negative species like Escherichia coli behind urinary tract infections. The addition of a β-lactamase inhibitor, clavulanic acid, further expands coverage against resistant pathogens.

While resistance has emerged, amoxicillin retains efficacy against key respiratory tract, skin, and soft tissue infections. It is considered a first-line antibiotic for otitis media, sinusitis, and pharyngitis. The World Health Organization deems amoxicillin an "Access" antibiotic for its importance on their Essential Medicines List.

Amoxicillin is also preferred over other broad-spectrum antibiotics when possible due to its safety profile. While it can cause diarrhea and allergic reactions, risks of clotting, kidney injury or liver toxicity are lower compared to alternatives. Amoxicillin is pregnancy category B, considered safe during expectant mothers.

Still, researchers continue improving amoxicillin's pharmacokinetic properties. Newer tablet formulations utilize specialized coatings for timed or extended release. Combining amoxicillin with beta-lactamase inhibitors like clavulanic acid expands coverage of resistant bacteria. Such innovations aim to prolong amoxicillin's clinical lifespan.

Continuous research also examines amoxicillin's emerging uses beyond infectious disease. Recent studies suggest amoxicillin could deplete harmful bacteria in the gut microbiome linked to obesity, diabetes, even dementia. As science reveals new roles of gut flora, amoxicillin may find additional purpose.

Over six decades since its discovery, amoxicillin remains a foundational antibiotic agent improving global public health, especially among children in the developing world. As a well-tolerated, cost-effective therapy, amoxicillin continues filling a vital place in medicine's arsenal against infectious disease.

Mechanisms of Action

The beta-lactam ring is the cornerstone of its mechanism of action. Amoxicillin belongs to the penicillin class of beta-lactam antibiotics. Like other beta-lactams, amoxicillin works by inhibiting bacterial cell wall synthesis, leading to cell death and stopping infection. However, the beta-lactam ring is also the site vulnerable to enzymatic degradation by bacterial beta-lactamases. This is why Amoxicillin is often combined with clavulanic acid, a beta-lactamase inhibitor, in formulations known as co-amoxiclav to counteract this resistance mechanism.

Bacteria produce a mesh-like cell wall that maintains their structure and integrity against the high osmotic pressure inside the cell. The main component of this rigid cell wall is peptidoglycan, composed of glycan strands cross-linked by short peptide chains.

Penicillin and its derivatives, including amoxicillin, work by binding to transpeptidase enzymes called penicillin-binding proteins (PBPs) that build the bacterial cell wall. Amoxicillin's chemical structure resembles the end segment of the peptidoglycan peptide chain.

When amoxicillin binds to PBPs, it blocks the cross-linking activity of these enzymes. This prevents incorporation of new peptidoglycan subunits into the existing cell wall. As a result, the cell wall weakens and osmotic pressure causes the bacterium to burst and die.

Amoxicillin is considered a broad-spectrum antibiotic because it inhibits multiple PBP enzymes found in both Gram-positive and Gram-negative bacteria. It has affinity for PBPs 1A, 1B, 2, and 3 which are essential transpeptidases found across many species.

By binding these targets, amoxicillin is bactericidal against key pathogens like Streptococcus pneumoniae, Haemophilus influenzae, and Moraxella catarrhalis that cause respiratory infections. It also kills Neisseria gonorrhoeae, the causative agent of gonorrhea.

Amoxicillin's spectrum extends to common Gram-negative bacteria like Escherichia coli, Klebsiella pneumoniae, Salmonella, Shigella, and Enterobacter. Such activity makes amoxicillin useful for urinary tract, gastrointestinal, and intra-abdominal infections where these bacteria predominate.

However, amoxicillin has limitations. Some species like Pseudomonas aeruginosa, a common hospital pathogen, lacks PBP targets sensitive to amoxicillin. Amoxicillin also cannot cross the outer membrane of certain Gram-negative bacteria, further restricting its spectrum.

Resistance arises when bacteria acquire mutations altering PBPs enough that amoxicillin can no longer bind them effectively. Bacteria may also acquire genes encoding β-lactamase enzymes that directly destroy amoxicillin before it reaches its targets.

Combining amoxicillin with a β-lactamase inhibitor like clavulanic acid protects the drug from enzymatic breakdown, overcoming some resistant strains. But PBP mutations still limit amoxicillin in treating emerging drug-resistant infections.

Understanding the specific PBP interactions and resistance mechanisms of amoxicillin guides researchers toward designing improved semi-synthetic penicillins. Structure-activity experiments reveal ways to enhance target affinity while evading resistance factors.

Future aminopenicillin development may involve modifying the acyl R-group side chain to optimize binding to critical transpeptidases like PBP2x in S. pneumoniae. Such innovations could restore activity against resistant respiratory pathogens.

After over 50 years of use, amoxicillin remains a foundational beta-lactam antibiotic targeting the penicillin-binding proteins and cell wall synthesis of both common Gram-positive and Gram-negative bacteria. Continued research on its structure and mechanism aims to preserve amoxicillin's efficacy against evolving bacteria.

The chemical structure also has implications for its manufacturing process. Being a semi-synthetic antibiotic,

Amoxicillin is prepared by modifying naturally occurring compounds, ensuring a high degree of purity and effectiveness. Rigorous quality control measures are applied during its manufacturing to guarantee that the final product meets the pharmacopeial standards for medical use.

Understanding the mechanism of action of Amoxicillin is critical for both healthcare providers and patients, as it informs proper usage, dosage, and even the limitations of this antibiotic. At its core, Amoxicillin is a bactericidal agent, meaning it kills bacteria rather than merely inhibiting their growth.

The primary target of Amoxicillin is the bacterial cell wall, a complex structure that provides rigidity and protection to the bacterial cell. Unlike human cells, bacterial cells have a thick wall made of a substance called peptidoglycan. Amoxicillin interferes with the synthesis of peptidoglycan, leading to a weakened cell wall that is unable to maintain its structural integrity. This causes the bacterial cell to burst and die, especially when it tries to divide and grow.

The beta-lactam ring in the chemical structure of Amoxicillin plays a vital role in its antibacterial activity. This ring mimics a component of the bacterial cell wall, deceiving bacterial enzymes called transpeptidases (or penicillin-binding proteins). These enzymes are tricked into binding with Amoxicillin instead of the peptidoglycan precursors, leading to faulty cell wall synthesis.

Amoxicillin is considered a broad-spectrum antibiotic, effective against a wide range of Gram-positive and some Gram-negative bacteria. However, it is not a panacea for all bacterial infections. Some bacteria produce enzymes called beta-lactamases that can break down the beta-lactam ring, rendering Amoxicillin ineffective. This is why Amoxicillin is often administered in combination with beta-lactamase inhibitors like clavulanic acid, as mentioned in the previous section on chemical structure.

Amoxicillin's excellent oral bioavailability means that it is well-absorbed from the gastrointestinal tract, reaching peak plasma concentrations within one to two hours of administration. It is distributed widely throughout the body, making it effective for treating infections in various tissues and organs. Unlike some other antibiotics, Amoxicillin is not extensively metabolized in the liver, and a majority of the drug is excreted unchanged in the urine. This also means that it has a relatively short half-life, requiring multiple doses per day for sustained antibacterial activity.

While Amoxicillin is highly effective, misuse can lead to bacterial resistance. Overuse, underuse, or improper dosage can result in the survival of some bacteria, which may develop mechanisms to counteract the drug. This is a growing concern in the medical community and underlines the importance of using antibiotics like Amoxicillin responsibly.

In summary, the mechanism of action of Amoxicillin is a well-orchestrated process that targets the fundamental biology of bacterial cells. Understanding this mechanism is essential for the effective and responsible use of this antibiotic, as it informs proper dosage and administration, and helps both healthcare providers and patients to appreciate its strengths and limitations.

Comparing Amoxicillin to Other Antibiotics

As an aminopenicillin antibiotic, amoxicillin is closely related to other penicillin derivatives but has properties distinguishing it from cephalosporins and other drug classes. These differences inform clinical decisions when selecting the most appropriate antibiotic to treat specific infections.

Compared to penicillin G, the first penicillin discovered, amoxicillin has a broader spectrum of activity against Gram-negative bacteria due to better penetration of the outer cell membrane. It is also better absorbed orally than penicillin G.

However, other aminopenicillins like ampicillin are very similar to amoxicillin. Ampicillin has a near identical spectrum of activity, covering the same range of Gram-positive and Gram-negative pathogens. The two drugs have similar absorption and pharmacokinetics.

The main advantage of amoxicillin over ampicillin is better tolerability, with less gastrointestinal distress like diarrhea. Amoxicillin also has slightly higher bioavailability when taken by mouth compared to ampicillin. Some bacteria have developed specific resistance to ampicillin but not amoxicillin.

Methicillin and other penicillinase-resistant penicillins are unaffected by beta-lactamase enzymes that hydrolyze amoxicillin. This makes them drugs of choice for serious Staphylococcus aureus infections. Amoxicillin has little intrinsic activity against Pseudomonas aeruginosa compared to piperacillin.

Cephalosporins like cefuroxime, cefpodoxime and cefdinir cover a similar spectrum as amoxicillin. However, some bacteria resistant to amoxicillin and other penicillins remain susceptible to certain cephalosporins and vice versa. Rotating between drug classes helps prevent resistance.

Fluoroquinolones like ciprofloxacin and levofloxacin are broad-spectrum alternatives for treating many common bacterial infections. However, growing fluoroquinolone resistance and side effects like tendonitis limit their use compared to relatively safe amoxicillin.

Macrolides such as azithromycin and clarithromycin are preferred over amoxicillin for atypical respiratory pathogens like Mycoplasma pneumoniae and Chlamydophila pneumoniae. The combination of a macrolide and amoxicillin provides empiric coverage when diagnosing pneumonia.

Clindamycin is another option for lung infections but covers a narrower spectrum. Tetracyclines like doxycycline have reduced activity compared to amoxicillin for key pathogens causing sinusitis, otitis media, and tonsillitis.

For intra-abdominal infections involving anaerobes like Bacteroides, alternatives like clindamycin or metronidazole may be used in combination with amoxicillin to ensure adequate coverage. Similarly, agents with anti-Pseudomonal coverage supplement amoxicillin when treating severe hospital-acquired infections.

Compared to sulfonamides like Bactrim, amoxicillin retains efficacy against most Gram-negative Enterobacterales that have grown resistant to older drugs. Amoxicillin is also not associated with severe hypersensitivity reactions that limit sulfonamide use.

In summary, while other drug classes have a place in therapy, amoxicillin remains one of the safest, most versatile first-line antibiotics for common outpatient infections. It is favored as an empiric therapy when the causative bacteria is unknown but broad-spectrum coverage is desired.

Knowing the overlap, gaps, benefits, and risks of amoxicillin compared to other antibiotic classes aids providers in selecting the optimal drug for each infection scenario. However, amoxicillin continues to serve a pivotal role across all age groups given its longevity of efficacy combined with its mild side effect profile.

.

TYPES OF INFECTIONS TREATABLE WITH AMOXICILLIN

Amoxicillin is a versatile antibiotic that is effective against a wide variety of bacterial infections. Its broad-spectrum activity makes it a go-to option for healthcare providers in treating multiple conditions. Below are some of the primary infections where Amoxicillin has proven to be particularly effective.

Treating Pneumonia with Amoxicillin

Pneumonia is a severe respiratory condition characterized by inflammation of the air sacs, or alveoli, in the lungs. It is a leading cause of hospitalization and death worldwide, particularly among children and the elderly. Various pathogens can cause pneumonia, including bacteria, viruses, and fungi. Among bacterial causes, Streptococcus pneumoniae is the most common culprit, and Amoxicillin is often the first-line treatment for community-acquired pneumonia. This chapter aims to provide an in-depth understanding of how Amoxicillin can be used to treat pneumonia effectively.

Pneumonia can present with a variety of symptoms, ranging from mild to severe. Common symptoms include cough, fever, chills, and difficulty breathing. The condition can be categorized based on the setting in which it was acquired—community-acquired or hospital-acquired—and the pathogens involved. Bacterial pneumonia is often more severe than viral pneumonia and requires prompt treatment with antibiotics.

Risk Factors

Several factors can increase the risk of developing pneumonia, including:

- Age: Infants and the elderly are more susceptible.

- Smoking: Smokers are at a higher risk compared to non-smokers.
- Chronic conditions: Conditions like asthma, COPD, and diabetes can make one more susceptible to pneumonia.
- Immunosuppression: Individuals with weakened immune systems are at higher risk.

Why Amoxicillin?

Amoxicillin is a broad-spectrum antibiotic, making it effective against a wide range of bacteria. It has an excellent safety profile and is well-tolerated, with few side effects. Its efficacy against Streptococcus pneumoniae, the leading cause of community-acquired bacterial pneumonia, makes it a first-line treatment option.

As discussed in previous chapters, Amoxicillin works by inhibiting bacterial cell wall synthesis. This is particularly effective against Streptococcus pneumoniae, which has a thick cell wall made of peptidoglycan. By interfering with the enzymes responsible for cell wall synthesis, Amoxicillin weakens the bacteria, causing it to burst and die.

The dosage of Amoxicillin for treating pneumonia varies depending on several factors, including the severity of the condition, patient age, and presence of other medical conditions. A typical adult dosage may range from 500 mg to 1 gram every 8 to 12 hours. For children, the dosage is often calculated based on body weight.

The duration of treatment also varies but is typically between 5 to 14 days. It is crucial to complete the entire course of treatment, even if symptoms improve before the medication is finished. Failure to complete the treatment can lead to bacterial resistance, making the bacteria harder to treat in the future.

While Amoxicillin is generally well-tolerated, it can cause some side effects, such as gastrointestinal issues like diarrhea, nausea, and vomiting. Less commonly, it can cause allergic reactions, so it's essential to inform your healthcare provider if you have a history of allergies to penicillin or other antibiotics.

Special Considerations

- Pregnancy and Breastfeeding: Amoxicillin is considered safe during pregnancy and breastfeeding but consult your healthcare provider for tailored advice.

- Co-existing Conditions: For patients with renal or liver impairment, the dosage may need to be adjusted.

Regular monitoring is crucial when treating pneumonia with Amoxicillin. This includes regular medical check-ups and, in some cases, additional tests like chest X-rays or blood tests to monitor the infection's progression.

Pneumonia is a severe respiratory infection that requires prompt and effective treatment. Amoxicillin serves as a first-line treatment for bacterial pneumonia, particularly that caused by Streptococcus pneumoniae. Its broad-spectrum activity, combined with an excellent safety profile and various administration options, make it a drug of choice for this condition. However, responsible use is critical to prevent the development of antibiotic-resistant strains of bacteria.

By understanding the ins and outs of treating pneumonia with Amoxicillin, healthcare providers and patients alike can contribute to better treatment outcomes and the responsible use of this valuable antibiotic.

Treating Urinary Tract Infections with Amoxicillin

Urinary tract infections (UTIs) are one of the most frequently encountered infections in healthcare, affecting millions globally each year. While UTIs can affect anyone, they are notably more prevalent among women. The infection can occur in any part of the urinary system: kidneys, bladder, urethra, and ureters. Amoxicillin, often in combination with clavulanic acid, has been a cornerstone in treating bacterial UTIs. This chapter aims to offer an in-depth understanding of the role of Amoxicillin in treating various types of UTIs.

Understanding Urinary Tract Infections

Urinary tract infections can manifest in different forms and severities. The infections are generally categorized based on the region of the urinary tract they affect and the complexities related to the infection. UTIs can affect any part of the urinary system, which includes the kidneys, bladder, ureters, and urethra. Symptoms often include frequent urination, a burning sensation during urination, cloudy urine, and lower abdominal pain.

Types of UTIs

Cystitis: This is a bladder infection and is the most common type of UTI. It's primarily caused by E. coli but can also be due to other bacteria.

Urethritis: This infection affects the urethra and can be caused by both bacterial and viral pathogens. Bacterial causes include E. coli and some sexually transmitted bacteria like gonorrhea and chlamydia.

Pyelonephritis: A kidney infection that is often a progression from a lower UTI. It can be severe and requires immediate treatment. E. coli is the most common bacterial cause.

Asymptomatic Bacteriuria: Presence of bacteria in the urine without symptoms. This is often found in pregnant women and may require treatment to prevent complications.

Risk Factors

Several risk factors can predispose individuals to UTIs:

- **Gender and Anatomy:** Women are at a higher risk due to shorter urethras.
- **Sexual Activity:** Sexual intercourse, especially with multiple partners, increases the risk.

- **Age:** UTIs are common in postmenopausal women and older men.
- **Catheter Use:** Long-term use of urinary catheters

Why Amoxicillin for UTIs?

Amoxicillin is a broad-spectrum antibiotic effective against a variety of bacteria, including E. coli, Staphylococcus saprophyticus, and Proteus mirabilis, commonly implicated in UTIs. The drug's pharmacokinetic properties, such as high oral bioavailability and effective concentrations in urine, make it a suitable choice for treating UTIs.

Amoxicillin's effectiveness against UTIs is attributed to its ability to inhibit bacterial cell wall synthesis. This action disrupts the bacteria's integrity, leading to cell death, particularly effective for gram-positive bacteria and some gram-negative bacteria when combined with clavulanic acid.

Dosage and Administration

Proper dosing is crucial for effective treatment. The dosage varies depending on several factors, including the type of UTI, patient age, and kidney function.

For Cystitis: Adults typically take 250-500 mg every 8 hours. For children, a weight-based dose ranging from 20-40 mg/kg/day divided into 2-3 doses is standard.

For Pyelonephritis: A higher dose is generally recommended, often 500 mg every 8 hours in adults.

For Urethritis and Asymptomatic Bacteriuria: Dosage generally aligns with that of cystitis but may be adjusted based on the specific bacteria involved.

Duration of Treatment

The length of antibiotic treatment varies:
Cystitis: 3-7 days
Pyelonephritis: At least 7-14 days
Urethritis and Asymptomatic Bacteriuria: Duration depends on clinical judgment and patient response.

Side Effects and Precautions

Common side effects include gastrointestinal disturbances like diarrhea and nausea. Less commonly, allergic reactions can occur. Always inform your healthcare provider of any allergies or other medications you are taking.

Special Considerations

Pregnancy: Amoxicillin is generally considered safe but consult your healthcare provider for personalized advice.

Elderly Patients: Dose adjustment may be required due to altered kidney function.

Patients with Kidney Impairment: Reduced dosage and/or extended dosing intervals may be necessary.

Amoxicillin, especially when combined with clavulanic acid, is a potent antibiotic for treating various types of UTIs. From cystitis to pyelonephritis, its broad spectrum of activity and excellent bioavailability make it a preferred choice. However, responsible use is crucial to avoid the development of antibiotic resistance. Always consult a healthcare provider for a diagnosis and treatment plan tailored to your condition.

Treating Otitis Media with Amoxicillin

Otitis media, commonly known as a middle ear infection, is a prevalent condition, especially among children. The infection can cause significant discomfort, manifesting as ear pain, hearing difficulties, and sometimes fever. While viral infections can lead to otitis media, bacterial causes often require antibiotic treatment. Amoxicillin is the first-line treatment for bacterial otitis media due to its efficacy, safety, and palatability in pediatric formulations. This chapter aims to provide a comprehensive, in-depth look at the role of Amoxicillin in managing otitis media.

Understanding Otitis Media

Otitis media is an inflammation or infection of the middle ear, the area behind the eardrum. The condition can be acute or chronic, and it can be categorized further based on its characteristics and symptoms.

Types of Otitis Media

- **Acute Otitis Media (AOM):** This is a sudden onset of symptoms, often following a respiratory infection. It is more common in children.

- **Otitis Media with Effusion (OME):** This type involves fluid accumulation in the middle ear without signs of infection. It can occur after AOM or independently.

- **Chronic Otitis Media:** This is a long-standing infection or inflammation of the middle ear and can lead to complications if not treated.

Common Bacterial Pathogens

- **Streptococcus pneumoniae:** The most common bacterial cause of AOM.

- **Haemophilus influenzae:** Another frequent cause, especially in children.

- **Moraxella catarrhalis:** Less common but still a significant pathogen in otitis media.

Why Amoxicillin for Otitis Media?

Amoxicillin is particularly effective against the common bacteria causing otitis media. It has a broad spectrum of activity and reaches effective concentrations in the middle ear fluid, making it an ideal choice for treatment.

Amoxicillin works by inhibiting bacterial cell wall synthesis, which leads to bacterial cell death. This is effective for both gram-positive bacteria like Streptococcus pneumoniae and some gram-negative bacteria like Haemophilus influenzae when used in appropriate doses.

Dosage and Administration

The dosage of Amoxicillin for treating otitis media varies based on the severity of the condition, the age of the patient, and other health considerations.

- **For Acute Otitis Media in Children**: A high-dose regimen is often recommended, such as 80-90 mg/kg/day divided into two doses. This is because higher doses have been found to be more effective against resistant strains of bacteria.

- **For Adults**: A standard dosage might range from 500 mg to 875 mg every 12 hours, depending on the severity and the causative bacteria.

- **For Chronic Otitis Media**: The treatment may require longer courses, often exceeding two weeks, and may include other treatment modalities such as surgical intervention.

Duration of Treatment

- **Acute Otitis Media**: Usually 5-10 days, depending on age and severity.

- Otitis Media with Effusion: Treatment duration depends on the persistence of symptoms and may require a different approach, including watchful waiting.

- Chronic Otitis Media: Prolonged treatment often exceeding two weeks, sometimes requiring surgical drainage.

Side Effects and Precautions

Amoxicillin is generally well-tolerated, but side effects can include:

- **Gastrointestinal Issues:** Such as diarrhea and nausea.

- **Allergic Reactions:** Rashes and, rarely, more severe allergic responses.

Special Considerations

- **Children:** Pediatric formulations are available, and the drug is generally well-tolerated in children.

- **Pregnancy and Breastfeeding:** Generally considered safe but consult your healthcare provider for a tailored treatment plan.

Otitis media is a common condition that can significantly affect quality of life, especially in children. Amoxicillin stands as a first-line treatment option due to its efficacy against common causative bacteria, excellent safety profile, and general tolerability. As with any antibiotic, responsible use is crucial to minimize the risk of bacterial resistance, making it vital to follow the healthcare provider's guidelines closely.

Treating Tooth Infections with Amoxicillin

Tooth infections, often referred to as dental abscesses or periapical abscesses, are common but potentially severe conditions that can lead to systemic complications if left untreated. These infections can occur in different parts of the tooth and surrounding tissues, causing symptoms like pain, swelling, and fever. Amoxicillin, often used as a first-line treatment for dental infections, is chosen for its broad-spectrum antimicrobial activity, excellent oral absorption, and general safety profile. This chapter aims to provide an exhaustive overview of using Amoxicillin in treating various types of tooth infections.

Understanding Tooth Infections

Tooth infections result from bacterial invasion into the dental pulp, the innermost part of the tooth, often due to cavities, cracked teeth, or gum disease. These infections can spread to surrounding tissues, leading to abscess formation.

Types of Tooth Infections

-   Periapical Abscess: An infection at the tip of the root of a tooth.

- Periodontal Abscess: An infection in the gums surrounding a tooth.

- Pericoronitis: Infection surrounding a partially erupted or impacted wisdom tooth.

Common Causative Agents

- Anaerobes: Such as Fusobacterium, Prevotella, and Peptostreptococcus species, are the most common bacteria in dental abscesses.

- Aerobes: Streptococcus species are also frequently involved.

Why Amoxicillin for Tooth Infections?

Amoxicillin is highly effective against the bacteria commonly found in dental abscesses. It has good oral bioavailability, ensuring that effective concentrations are reached at the site of infection. Additionally, its broad-spectrum action makes it suitable for polymicrobial infections, which are common in dental cases.

Amoxicillin disrupts the bacterial cell wall synthesis, leading to bacterial cell lysis and death. This action is especially crucial for anaerobic bacteria, which are commonly found in dental abscesses.

Dosage and Administration

Dosing strategies for dental infections vary based on the severity of the infection and patient-specific factors. However, typical dosing guidelines include:

- **Adults**: 500 mg every 8 to 12 hours, often for 3 to 7 days.

- **Children**: Dosing is usually weight-based, with a common range being 20-40 mg/kg/day divided into three doses.

Duration of Treatment

- Acute Dental Abscess: Treatment often lasts for 3 to 7 days but may be extended if the infection is severe or complications arise.

- Chronic or Recurrent Infections: May require longer treatment durations and possibly surgical intervention.

Side Effects and Precautions

The most common side effects are gastrointestinal, including nausea and diarrhea. Allergic reactions, although rare, can occur and range from mild skin rashes to severe anaphylactic reactions.

Special Considerations

- **Patients with Penicillin Allergy**: Alternative antibiotics like clindamycin may be considered.

- **Pregnancy and Breastfeeding**: Amoxicillin is generally considered safe but consult your healthcare provider for personalized advice.

- **Renal Impairment**: Dose adjustments may be necessary.

Tooth infections can be debilitating and potentially dangerous if left untreated. Amoxicillin offers a highly effective, safe, and well-tolerated treatment option for various types of dental infections. However, it's crucial to use this antibiotic responsibly and under medical supervision to mitigate the risks of antibiotic resistance and ensure optimal treatment outcomes.

Treating Skin Infections with Amoxicillin

Skin infections, including conditions like cellulitis, impetigo, and abscesses, can range from mild annoyances to severe conditions requiring hospitalization. While a variety of bacteria can cause skin infections, Staphylococcus aureus and Streptococcus pyogenes are the most common culprits. Amoxicillin, with its broad-spectrum activity and excellent pharmacokinetic properties, is frequently used to treat bacterial skin infections. This chapter aims to provide an exhaustive, in-depth view of how Amoxicillin can be employed to manage various skin infections effectively.

Understanding Skin Infections

Skin infections can manifest in various forms, each with its own set of symptoms, causes, and treatment approaches. These infections may be superficial, affecting just the epidermis, or more severe, extending into deeper layers of the skin and even the bloodstream.

Types of Skin Infections

- **Cellulitis:** A deep skin infection affecting the dermis and subcutaneous tissue, often caused by Streptococcus or Staphylococcus bacteria.

- **Impetigo:** A highly contagious superficial infection commonly seen in children, often caused by Staphylococcus aureus or Streptococcus pyogenes.

- **Skin Abscesses:** Collections of pus within the dermis and deeper skin tissues, often caused by Staphylococcus aureus, including MRSA (Methicillin-Resistant Staphylococcus Aureus).

Why Amoxicillin for Skin Infections?

Amoxicillin is effective against a range of bacteria commonly responsible for skin infections. Its high oral bioavailability ensures effective concentrations at the site of infection, and its good safety profile makes it suitable for both adults and children.

Amoxicillin targets the bacterial cell wall, inhibiting its synthesis and thus causing bacterial cell death. This is especially effective against gram-positive bacteria like Staphylococcus and Streptococcus, which are commonly involved in skin infections.

Dosage and Administration

The dosage regimen for treating skin infections with Amoxicillin is tailored to the type and severity of the infection, as well as patient-specific factors like age and kidney function.

- **For Cellulitis:** Adults may be prescribed 500 mg every 8 to 12 hours for 7 to 14 days, depending on the severity.

- **For Impetigo**: Children may receive a weight-based dosage, such as 25 to 50 mg/kg/day divided into two or three doses for about a week.

- **For Skin Abscesses**: Treatment often involves drainage, but Amoxicillin can be used as adjunctive therapy, particularly if the abscess is large or complicated.

Duration of Treatment

-   **Cellulitis**: Generally 7 to 14 days, depending on patient response and severity.

-   **Impetigo**: Usually 7 days, unless complications occur.

-   **Skin Abscesses**: Duration varies, especially if surgical intervention is required.

Side Effects and Precautions

Common side effects are similar to those with other uses of Amoxicillin and include gastrointestinal symptoms like nausea and diarrhea. Allergic reactions are rare but can be severe.

Special Considerations

- **MRSA Infections**: Amoxicillin is not effective against MRSA and alternative antibiotics like clindamycin or trimethoprim-sulfamethoxazole may be used.

- **Penicillin Allergy**: Alternatives like clindamycin or macrolides may be considered.

- **Pregnancy and Breastfeeding**: Amoxicillin is generally considered safe but consult your healthcare provider for personalized advice.

Skin infections can range from mild to severe and may lead to complications if not adequately treated. Amoxicillin provides a potent tool in the treatment of various skin infections, due to its broad-spectrum efficacy, excellent bioavailability, and favorable safety profile. However, appropriate dosing and duration are crucial, and the antibiotic should be used responsibly to mitigate the risk of bacterial resistance.

Treating Salmonella Infections with Amoxicillin

Salmonella infections, commonly known as salmonellosis, are caused by bacteria belonging to the genus Salmonella. These infections are often associated with foodborne outbreaks but can also be contracted through direct contact with infected animals or people. While most cases of salmonellosis are self-limiting and don't require antibiotic treatment, severe or complicated cases may necessitate the use of antibiotics like Amoxicillin. This chapter aims to offer a comprehensive, in-depth understanding of the role of Amoxicillin in treating salmonellosis.

Understanding Salmonella Infections

Salmonella infections typically affect the gastrointestinal tract but can also lead to more severe conditions like typhoid fever, caused by specific Salmonella serotypes. The symptoms usually include diarrhea, fever, abdominal cramps, and vomiting.

Types of Salmonella Infections

-   **Non-typhoidal Salmonellosis**: Caused by various Salmonella serotypes, typically leading to gastrointestinal symptoms.

- **Typhoid Fever**: Caused by Salmonella Typhi or Salmonella Paratyphi, this is a more severe form of infection that can affect various organs.

Why Amoxicillin for Salmonella?

Amoxicillin is effective against Salmonella bacteria, including Salmonella Typhi, making it a treatment option for both non-typhoidal salmonellosis and typhoid fever. Its good oral bioavailability ensures effective concentrations in the gastrointestinal tract and bloodstream, where these bacteria are commonly found.

Amoxicillin inhibits bacterial cell wall synthesis, resulting in the death of bacterial cells. Given that Salmonella is a gram-negative bacterium, Amoxicillin's action on the bacterial cell wall is particularly crucial for the treatment of salmonellosis.

Dosage and Administration

The dosage of Amoxicillin for treating Salmonella infections varies based on the severity of the infection and patient-specific factors such as age and kidney function.

- **For Non-typhoidal Salmonellosis**: In severe cases requiring antibiotic treatment, adults may be prescribed 500 mg every 8 hours for 5-7 days.

- **For Typhoid Fever**: The regimen is more prolonged, often involving 500 mg every 8 hours for 14-21 days.

Duration of Treatment

- **Non-typhoidal Salmonellosis**: Usually 5-7 days, depending on the severity and patient response.

- **Typhoid Fever**: Typically requires a longer course of treatment, often 14-21 days, to ensure complete eradication of the bacteria.

Side Effects and Precautions

Common side effects include gastrointestinal disturbances like nausea and diarrhea. Allergic reactions are also possible but are generally rare.

Special Considerations

- **Antibiotic Resistance**: The rise of antibiotic-resistant Salmonella strains is a growing concern. Therefore, antibiotic susceptibility testing is often recommended.

- **Pregnancy and Breastfeeding**: Amoxicillin is generally considered safe, but consult your healthcare provider for personalized advice.

- **Children and Elderly**: Dosing adjustments may be required based on age and renal function.

Salmonella infections can range from mild, self-limiting gastrointestinal illnesses to severe conditions like typhoid fever. Amoxicillin serves as a useful antibiotic for treating severe or complicated cases of salmonellosis. Its broad-spectrum activity, high oral bioavailability, and general safety make it a viable treatment option. However, due to the increasing rates of antibiotic resistance, it is crucial to use Amoxicillin responsibly and usually only when deemed necessary by a healthcare provider.

DOSAGE AND ADMINISTRATION

The accurate dosage and correct administration of Amoxicillin are not merely a matter of following prescriptions but involve a nuanced understanding of pharmacokinetics and pharmacodynamics. This antibiotic, belonging to the penicillin class, is commonly used to treat a variety of bacterial infections, from skin and dental infections to more severe conditions like pneumonia. This chapter aims to provide an exhaustive discussion of how to administer Amoxicillin effectively, based on various considerations such as age, weight, type of infection, and individual health conditions.

General Guidelines

When prescribing Amoxicillin, healthcare providers usually start by considering the general dosing guidelines. These guidelines are based on extensive clinical trials and real-world experience but should always be tailored to individual patient needs. Standard adult dosages often range from 250 mg to 500 mg, taken every 8 hours. For children, the dose is typically calculated based on weight, often around 20 to 50 mg/kg divided into multiple doses per day. Amoxicillin comes in several forms, including oral capsules, tablets, chewable tablets, and liquid suspensions. Each form has its own set of guidelines:

- **Capsules and Tablets:** Usually taken with or without food every 8 to 12 hours, as prescribed.

- **Chewable Tablets:** Must be chewed before swallowing, not to be swallowed whole.

- **Liquid Suspension:** Must be shaken well before each use and measured with a medical-grade syringe or cup.

The route of administration is generally oral for most infections, but intravenous options are available for severe or hospital-treated conditions.

Importance of Adherence

One of the most critical aspects of antibiotic treatment is completing the full course, even if symptoms resolve earlier. Incomplete treatment can lead to bacterial resistance, a growing global health concern.

Dosage by Age and Weight

- **Adults**: The adult dosage typically ranges from 250 mg to 875 mg, administered every 8 to 12 hours. Severe infections like pneumonia may require the higher end of this range, and sometimes the addition of another antibiotic for a synergistic effect.

- **Children**: Pediatric dosing is generally calculated based on weight. The usual pediatric dosage ranges from 20 mg/kg/day to 50 mg/kg/day, divided into two or three doses. For example, in otitis media, higher doses up to 90 mg/kg/day may be used.

Adjustments for Special Populations

- **Elderly**: Reduced dosages may be required due to decreased renal function.

- **Renal Impairment**: Dosage adjustments are often needed due to decreased drug clearance.

Duration of Treatment

The treatment's duration can vary significantly based on the type of infection and its severity. For example:

- **Respiratory Tract Infections**: The standard treatment course is often 7 to 14 days but may extend up to 21 days for severe cases like bacterial pneumonia.

- **Urinary Tract Infections**: A shorter course of 3 to 7 days is generally effective for uncomplicated UTIs. However, pyelonephritis or complicated UTIs may require a 14-day course or longer.

- **Skin Infections**: The treatment duration typically ranges from 7 to 14 days but can extend further if the infection is severe or if surgical intervention is required.

It's crucial to complete the full antibiotic course as prescribed, even if symptoms improve, to ensure complete eradication of the bacterial pathogen and to minimize the risk of developing antibiotic resistance.

Monitoring and Follow-up

Patients on Amoxicillin should be closely monitored for treatment efficacy and potential side effects. Follow-up appointments and, in some cases, lab tests are crucial to ensure the infection has been fully eradicated and to catch any adverse effects early.

In conclusion, the dosage and administration of Amoxicillin are multi-faceted topics that require a tailored approach based on numerous variables. Incorrect dosing can lead not only to treatment failure but also contribute to the larger issue of antibiotic resistance. Therefore, it's crucial to consult healthcare providers for a personalized treatment plan and adhere strictly to the prescribed regimen.

POTENTIAL SIDE EFFECTS

W hile Amoxicillin is generally well-tolerated and effective for treating various bacterial infections, it is not devoid of potential side effects. Understanding these adverse effects, ranging from mild to severe, is crucial for safe and effective treatment. This chapter aims to provide an exhaustive, in-depth discussion on the possible side effects of Amoxicillin, encompassing common symptoms, serious adverse reactions, and drug interactions.

Common Side Effects

Amoxicillin, like many antibiotics, can cause a range of common side effects that usually do not require discontinuation of the medication:

- **Gastrointestinal Issues:** Nausea, vomiting, and diarrhea are the most commonly reported side effects. Taking the medication with food can sometimes alleviate these symptoms.

- **Oral and Vaginal Thrush:** The antibiotic can disrupt the natural flora of the mouth and vagina, leading to fungal overgrowth known as thrush.

- **Skin Rash:** Mild skin rashes are not uncommon and usually resolve after discontinuation.

Management of Common Side Effects

- **Hydration:** Maintaining adequate fluid intake can help manage diarrhea.

- **Probiotics:** These can help restore gut flora, although their efficacy is still under study.

- **Antifungal Medication:** May be prescribed for thrush.

Serious Side Effects

While rare, Amoxicillin can cause serious side effects that require immediate medical attention:

- **Allergic Reactions**: Allergic reactions to Amoxicillin can range from mild skin rashes to severe anaphylaxis. Patients with a known allergy to penicillin or other beta-lactam antibiotics are at higher risk and should avoid taking Amoxicillin. Cross-reactivity between penicillins and cephalosporins has also been reported, so caution is advised for patients with known allergies to other classes of antibiotics. In cases where an allergic reaction is suspected, treatment with Amoxicillin should be discontinued immediately, and alternative antibiotics should be considered.

- **Severe Diarrhea**: Caused by an overgrowth of the bacteria Clostridium difficile, this can lead to severe colitis.

- **Liver Dysfunction**: Elevated liver enzymes and jaundice have been reported but are generally reversible upon discontinuation.

Reporting and Management

Any severe or unexpected side effects should be promptly reported to healthcare providers. Depending on the symptom's severity, your doctor may adjust the dosage or switch to a different antibiotic.

DRUG INTERACTIONS

Amoxicillin is a versatile antibiotic, but its efficacy and safety can be influenced by interactions with other drugs. This is a critical area of concern for both healthcare providers and patients. Drug interactions can lead to a range of outcomes, from reduced effectiveness of the medication to increased risk of side effects or toxicity. Amoxicillin can interact with several other medications, impacting their efficacy or increasing the risk of side effects.

Drugs to Avoid

Certain medications should be used cautiously or avoided altogether when taking Amoxicillin. For example:

- **Oral Contraceptives**: Amoxicillin and other antibiotics have been reported to reduce the effectiveness of oral contraceptives, although the evidence is somewhat mixed. The proposed mechanism involves changes in the gut flora responsible for re-circulating estrogen, an active component of most oral contraceptives. This interaction can lead to reduced levels of circulating estrogen and thus, a decreased contraceptive effect. Women using oral contraceptives should be advised to use an additional form of contraception during the course of Amoxicillin and for some time afterward. The ramifications of unintended pregnancies can be significant and can lead to a cascade of psychological, social, and medical issues.

- **Allopurinol**: Concurrent use can increase the risk of allergic skin reactions.

- **Methotrexate**: Another significant interaction occurs with methotrexate, a drug commonly used for treating certain types of cancer and autoimmune conditions like rheumatoid arthritis. Methotrexate is primarily excreted through the kidneys, and Amoxicillin can interfere with this process. The antibiotic can reduce the renal clearance of methotrexate, leading to increased levels of the drug in the bloodstream and potential toxicity. Methotrexate toxicity can manifest in several ways, including bone marrow suppression, liver toxicity, and severe mucositis. For patients on both medications, close monitoring of methotrexate blood levels and comprehensive assessments of renal function are essential. Dosage adjustments or even temporary discontinuation of one or both drugs may be warranted based on the clinical scenario.

- **Anticoagulants:** One of the most critical classes of drugs to be cautious of when using Amoxicillin is anticoagulants, particularly warfarin. Warfarin's primary mechanism of action involves inhibiting the synthesis of vitamin K-dependent clotting factors. Amoxicillin can alter the gut microbiota responsible for synthesizing vitamin K. This interaction can potentiate the anticoagulant effect of warfarin, increasing the risk of bleeding events. It's not just about spontaneous bleeding; even minor injuries can lead to significant blood loss when such an interaction occurs. The implications are even more severe for patients who are already at an elevated risk for bleeding, such as those with liver diseases, a history of gastrointestinal ulcers, or concomitant use of other medications that increase bleeding risk like aspirin or certain antiplatelet drugs. Therefore, patients on warfarin who are prescribed Amoxicillin should be closely monitored through frequent checks of their

international normalized ratio (INR), a laboratory test
that measures blood clotting.

Safe Combinations

- **Clavulanic Acid:**
  Often combined with Amoxicillin to enhance its
  spectrum of activity and counteract bacterial resistance
  mechanisms.

- **Antacids and Amoxicillin:**
  One common concern for patients on antibiotics is
  gastrointestinal discomfort, which often leads to the
  use of antacids. Fortunately, antacids generally do not
  interfere with the pharmacokinetics of Amoxicillin.
  This is unlike certain other antibiotics like
  tetracyclines, whose absorption can be significantly
  reduced by antacids. Therefore, if a patient on
  Amoxicillin experiences mild gastrointestinal
  symptoms, antacids can be safely used. However,
  healthcare providers should still be cautious and
  monitor for any unusual symptoms or lack of efficacy
  in the antibiotic treatment.

- **Pain Relievers:**
  Common over-the-counter pain relievers like
  acetaminophen and ibuprofen are generally safe to use
  with Amoxicillin. These medications do not typically
  interfere with the antibiotic's efficacy or increase the
  risk of adverse effects. However, caution should be
  exercised in patients with liver or kidney issues or those

taking other medications that could interact with these pain relievers.

- **Antihypertensive Medications:**
  High blood pressure is a prevalent condition, and many patients on antibiotics like Amoxicillin may also be taking antihypertensive medications. The good news is that most antihypertensive classes, including beta-blockers, ACE inhibitors, and calcium channel blockers, generally do not have significant interactions with Amoxicillin. These medications act on different physiological pathways that do not overlap with those of Amoxicillin, making them safe for co-administration. Nonetheless, it's always a good practice for healthcare providers to monitor blood pressure regularly to ensure that the antihypertensive medication remains effective.

- **Probiotics:**
  The use of probiotics alongside antibiotics is an area of growing interest. The rationale is to replenish the gut microbiota that may be disturbed by antibiotic treatment, thus potentially reducing side effects like diarrhea. Some studies suggest that certain strains of probiotics can be safely and effectively used alongside antibiotics, including Amoxicillin, to reduce gastrointestinal side effects. However, more research is needed in this area, and it's crucial to choose probiotics that have been well-studied and proven to be safe for use with antibiotics.

In conclusion, while drug interactions are a significant concern in modern medicine, many medications can be safely co-administered with Amoxicillin. Understanding these safe combinations allows healthcare providers to manage symptoms effectively, optimize treatment outcomes, and improve patient satisfaction and adherence. However, it's crucial to remember that even "safe" combinations should be regularly reviewed and monitored, especially in patients with multiple comorbidities or those on long-term medication regimens. Always consult with healthcare providers for the most accurate and personalized advice regarding medication side effects.

SPECIAL CONSIDERATIONS

The administration of antibiotics, including Amoxicillin, is a complex task that extends beyond merely following a prescription. Various factors, such as existing health conditions, age, and even life stages like pregnancy, can influence how this medication should be administered. This chapter aims to provide a detailed, comprehensive guide on these special considerations, designed to equip healthcare providers, patients, and caregivers with the necessary knowledge to make informed decisions.

Pregnancy and Breastfeeding

One of the most critical periods during which special considerations come into play is pregnancy. During these nine months, the body undergoes significant physiological changes that can affect how drugs like Amoxicillin are metabolized and utilized.

Safety Profile in Pregnancy

Amoxicillin is classified under Category B for pregnancy by the Food and Drug Administration (FDA), meaning animal reproduction studies have not indicated a risk to the fetus, but there are no adequate and well-controlled studies in pregnant women. In general, Amoxicillin is considered safe during all trimesters of pregnancy, but a thorough risk-benefit analysis is essential.

- **First Trimester:** During the early stages of pregnancy, organogenesis— the formation of the baby's organs— takes place. Although Amoxicillin is generally considered safe, it is crucial to weigh the risks and benefits carefully. The drug should only be used if the potential benefits justify the possible risks to the fetus.

- **Second and Third Trimesters:** As the fetus grows, so does its exposure to medications taken by the mother. During these stages, healthcare providers often continue to recommend Amoxicillin for bacterial infections that pose a more significant health risk to both the mother and fetus if left untreated.

Breastfeeding Considerations

Amoxicillin is excreted in breast milk but in minimal amounts. The American Academy of Pediatrics classifies Amoxicillin as compatible with breastfeeding. However, the nursing infant should be monitored for potential adverse effects, the most common of which include gastrointestinal disturbances like diarrhea or skin rashes.

- **Infant Monitoring**: While the risk is low, infants should be closely observed for any signs of adverse reactions. Symptoms to watch for include diarrhea, irritability, and unusual fussiness, which could theoretically be attributed to exposure to Amoxicillin through breast milk.

- **Maternal Health**: On the maternal side, it's also crucial to monitor for symptoms indicating an unresolved infection or antibiotic side effects. If the nursing mother experiences persistent symptoms, further evaluation and potential change in treatment may be required.

Pediatric and Geriatric Use

Pediatric Population

Amoxicillin is a frequently prescribed antibiotic for children due to its efficacy against a wide range of bacterial infections and its generally favorable safety profile. However, there are several considerations specific to pediatric patients:

- Weight-Based Dosing: Unlike adults, where a standard dose often suffices, pediatric dosing is usually calculated based on the child's weight. This approach aims to optimize the drug's efficacy while minimizing the risk of adverse effects.

- Liquid Formulations: Children who cannot swallow pills can take Amoxicillin in liquid form. However, this form must be properly measured using a medicine syringe or dropper to ensure accurate dosing.

- Taste and Compliance: The liquid form of Amoxicillin is flavored, but not all children find it palatable, posing a challenge for caregivers in ensuring compliance. Mixing the antibiotic with a small amount of food or drink can sometimes help, but consult a healthcare provider for advice tailored to your child's needs.

Geriatric Population

The geriatric population often presents a unique set of challenges in medication management, mainly due to comorbidities and the physiological changes associated with aging:

- Renal Function: Kidney function generally declines with age, affecting how drugs are eliminated from the body. As a result, older adults may require dosage adjustments to avoid potential toxicity.

- Polypharmacy: Many older adults are on multiple medications, increasing the risk of drug interactions. Careful medication reconciliation is necessary when adding a new antibiotic like Amoxicillin to the regimen.

Renal and Liver Impairment

Renal Impairment

Amoxicillin is primarily excreted through the kidneys, making renal function a critical factor in its dosing. Patients with impaired renal function are at higher risk for drug accumulation, potentially leading to toxicity.

- **Dosage Adjustment:** The typical adult dosage may need to be reduced, or the dosing interval extended, to avoid excessive drug levels in the bloodstream.

- **Monitoring:** Frequent monitoring, including kidney function tests and possibly blood levels of the drug, may be necessary to tailor the treatment appropriately.

Liver Impairment

While Amoxicillin is not primarily metabolized by the liver, liver dysfunction can still impact its safe use:

- **Caution in Hepatic Diseases:** In conditions like cirrhosis, the drug's pharmacokinetics might be altered. Though not commonly done, some healthcare providers may opt for liver function tests before and during treatment.

- **Potential for Hepatotoxicity**: Although rare, Amoxicillin can cause liver enzyme elevations and, in extreme cases, hepatic dysfunction. Patients with pre-existing liver conditions should be closely monitored during treatment.

RESISTANCE AND MISUSE OF ANTIBIOTICS

Antibiotic resistance is a pressing global health concern that compromises the ability to treat infectious diseases effectively. Amoxicillin, like all antibiotics, is susceptible to the development of resistance if misused. This chapter aims to provide an exhaustive, in-depth discussion on the rising issue of antibiotic resistance, focusing on its causes, implications, and how responsible Amoxicillin use can mitigate this problem.

The Growing Problem

The looming threat of antibiotic resistance is an issue that has captured the attention of healthcare professionals, policymakers, and researchers worldwide. As bacteria evolve to evade the drugs designed to kill them, our arsenal of effective treatments dwindles, leading to a crisis that could thrust medicine back into an era where even minor infections were often fatal.

One of the leading contributors to the crisis is the overuse and misuse of antibiotics. In many instances, antibiotics like Amoxicillin are prescribed for conditions that do not require them. For example, it's not uncommon for patients to expect antibiotics for viral infections like the common cold, against which these drugs are ineffective. Such misuse not only contributes to antibiotic resistance but also exposes patients to unnecessary risks of side effects.

Healthcare providers play a critical role in the responsible prescribing of antibiotics. The onus is on them to determine whether the symptoms presented indeed warrant antibiotic treatment. Often, this requires thorough diagnostic testing, such as bacterial cultures, to confirm the presence of a bacterial infection.

However, the healthcare system itself often pressures doctors into overprescribing. Whether due to time constraints in busy practices or the patient's insistence on receiving an antibiotic, healthcare providers may find it easier to prescribe an antibiotic "just in case," further fueling the problem of resistance.

Another significant issue is self-medication and the failure to complete antibiotic courses. Patients who don't finish their antibiotic courses contribute to the problem in two ways: first, by potentially not entirely clearing the infection, and second, by allowing bacteria to develop resistance to the drug. Incomplete courses offer a 'training ground' for bacteria to evolve and adapt, making them harder to kill in the future.

The use of antibiotics extends beyond human medicine. Agribusinesses often use these drugs to promote growth or prevent disease within livestock populations. This widespread use in animals contributes to the overall burden of antibiotic resistance, as resistant bacteria from animal populations can transfer to humans through the food chain, direct contact, or environmental spread.

The issue of antibiotic resistance is not confined to any single country or healthcare system. Resistant bacteria know no borders. An infection that becomes untreatable in one part of the world poses a risk everywhere else. International travel and trade mean that antibiotic resistance is a global problem requiring coordinated, international solutions.

The economic implications of antibiotic resistance are staggering. As infections become more challenging to treat, healthcare costs soar due to longer hospital stays, more intensive care, and the need for more expensive medications. The societal costs are equally daunting, impacting productivity due to increased illness and potential disability.

While the picture may seem grim, efforts are underway to combat antibiotic resistance. These include the development of new antibiotics, although this is a lengthy and expensive process. More promising are strategies aimed at better antibiotic stewardship: educating healthcare providers and the public, improving diagnostic testing to better identify bacterial infections, and implementing policies to reduce unnecessary antibiotic use, both in healthcare and agriculture.

In conclusion, the growing problem of antibiotic resistance is a complex issue with multiple contributing factors, from healthcare practices to agricultural usage. The consequences of this crisis are dire, affecting not just individual health but societal well-being and economic stability. Combating this issue requires a multi-faceted approach involving better education, improved diagnostic methods, and more responsible antibiotic use. Only through concerted, global efforts can we hope to stem the tide of this growing threat.

How to Use Antibiotics Responsibly

In an era where antibiotic resistance is a growing concern, the onus of using these lifesaving drugs responsibly falls on both healthcare providers and patients. Amoxicillin, a commonly prescribed antibiotic, is no exception to this. This section aims to delve deeply into the subject of responsible antibiotic use, focusing on accurate diagnosis, appropriate dosing, monitoring, and the role of education in mitigating the problem of resistance.

The first step in responsible antibiotic use is an accurate diagnosis. Infections can be caused by various pathogens, including bacteria, viruses, and fungi. Antibiotics like Amoxicillin are effective only against bacterial infections.

Diagnostic Tests

Various diagnostic tests can help determine the nature of the infection. These may include:

- **Culture Tests**: These are the gold standard for identifying bacterial infections. Samples from blood, urine, or other affected areas are cultured in a lab to identify the bacteria responsible for the infection.

- **Rapid Tests:** For some infections, rapid diagnostic tests, such as the rapid strep test for streptococcal pharyngitis, can provide quick results.

Challenges in Diagnosis

However, accurate diagnosis is often hindered by several factors:

- **Limited Access:** Not all healthcare settings have immediate access to advanced diagnostic tests.

- **Time Constraints:** Bacterial cultures can take time, and a rapid diagnosis is often needed, especially in acute cases.

- **Cost:** The cost of diagnostic tests can be prohibitive, leading healthcare providers to sometimes rely solely on clinical symptoms, which is not always reliable.

Appropriate Dosing

Once a bacterial infection is confirmed, the next step is determining the appropriate dosage of the antibiotic. Incorrect dosing can lead to treatment failure and contribute to antibiotic resistance. Some factors Influencing Dosing are:

- **Type of Infection:** The severity and location of the infection play a crucial role in dosing. For instance, severe or systemic infections may require higher doses compared to localized infections.

- **Patient-Specific Factors**: Age, weight, renal and liver function, and other co-morbidities are considered when prescribing antibiotics.

Healthcare providers must consider these factors carefully when prescribing antibiotics. Guidelines are available for many common bacterial infections, but these are not a substitute for clinical judgment. Ongoing training in antibiotic stewardship for healthcare providers is crucial in ensuring responsible prescribing.

Monitoring and Follow-Up

Regular monitoring during antibiotic treatment is essential for several reasons:

- **Assessing Effectiveness**: Follow-up appointments can help assess whether the antibiotic is effectively treating the infection.

- **Identifying Side Effects**: Monitoring can also catch potential side effects early, allowing for timely intervention.

Various methods can be used for monitoring, depending on the nature of the infection and the patient's overall health:

- **Clinical Assessment:** This involves a thorough physical examination and history-taking to assess the patient's response to treatment.

- **Laboratory Tests:** Repeat cultures, blood tests, or imaging studies may be needed, particularly for more severe or complicated infections.

Both healthcare providers and patients need to be educated about the responsible use of antibiotics. This education can take several forms:

- **Public Awareness Campaigns:** These aim to inform the general public about the dangers of antibiotic misuse.

- **Provider Training:** Ongoing training in antibiotic stewardship is crucial for healthcare providers to stay updated on best practices.

- **Patient Counseling:** Educating patients about the importance of completing their antibiotic course, even if they feel better, can help prevent resistance.

In conclusion, responsible antibiotic use is a multi-faceted issue that involves accurate diagnosis, appropriate dosing, regular monitoring, and comprehensive education. Each of these components plays a critical role in combating the growing threat of antibiotic resistance. By understanding and applying these principles, both healthcare providers and patients can contribute to a more sustainable use of antibiotics like Amoxicillin.

CASE STUDIES

The real-world implications of antibiotic use and misuse can be best understood through case studies. These narratives not only serve as cautionary tales but also as success stories that underline the importance of responsible antibiotic usage.

Success Stories

1. Patient A - The Case of Multi-Drug-Resistant Infection

A 35-year-old individual was admitted to the hospital with a high fever, chills, and severe abdominal pain. Initial tests were inconclusive, and the patient was initially treated with a broad-spectrum antibiotic while awaiting further test results.

After 48 hours, bacterial cultures revealed a multi-drug-resistant strain of E. coli affecting the gastrointestinal tract. The bacteria were sensitive to only a few antibiotics, including Amoxicillin.

The healthcare team promptly switched the treatment to a high-dose Amoxicillin regimen, administered intravenously due to the severity of the infection. The patient was also given supportive treatments, including fluids and electrolytes, to manage symptoms.

The patient initially showed signs of an allergic reaction, including a minor skin rash. An allergy panel was immediately conducted, which ruled out an Amoxicillin allergy, attributing the rash to the infection itself.

The patient adhered to a strict 14-day intravenous Amoxicillin treatment. Follow-up cultures and imaging studies showed that the infection had been completely eradicated. This case underscores the importance of accurate diagnosis, timely treatment switches, and the effective use of Amoxicillin even in multi-drug-resistant infections.

2. Patient B - Pediatric Case with Recurrent Otitis Media

A 7-year-old child had recurrent episodes of otitis media, causing significant discomfort and affecting school performance. Previous antibiotic treatments had been partially effective but failed to prevent recurrence.

A detailed medical history was taken, which revealed frequent episodes of upper respiratory tract infections. Audiometric tests showed a mild hearing loss, raising concerns about potential long-term complications.

The healthcare provider decided to switch the treatment plan to a weight-based, high-dose Amoxicillin regimen, along with a probiotic to balance gut flora affected by prolonged antibiotic use.

Ensuring adherence to the medication was a challenge due to the child's aversion to the taste of the antibiotic. A flavored Amoxicillin suspension was prescribed, and the parents were educated on the importance of completing the antibiotic course.

The child completed the full course of Amoxicillin. Subsequent audiometric tests showed improved hearing, and the child reported feeling better, with no new episodes of otitis media occurring in the following months. The case emphasizes the need for accurate diagnosis, individualized treatment, and the importance of patient education, particularly in pediatric cases.

Cautionary Tales

1. Patient X - The Misuse of Antibiotics for Viral Infections

A 50-year-old patient with a history of recurrent upper respiratory tract infections presented to the clinic with symptoms of fever, sore throat, and fatigue. Despite feeling unwell, the patient insisted on a prescription for Amoxicillin, believing it to be a "cure-all" based on past experiences.

The healthcare provider, pressed for time and swayed by the patient's insistence, prescribed Amoxicillin without conducting proper diagnostic tests. No bacterial cultures or rapid viral tests were done to confirm the nature of the infection.

The patient took the prescribed Amoxicillin course but saw no improvement in symptoms. Instead, the patient experienced gastrointestinal side effects, including diarrhea and abdominal pain. Upon returning to the clinic, further tests revealed that the infection was viral in nature, making the use of antibiotics inappropriate and ineffective.

This case highlights the dangers of patient-led antibiotic prescriptions and the importance of proper diagnostics. It shows how both healthcare providers and patients can contribute to antibiotic misuse, which ultimately led to ineffective treatment and avoidable side effects.

2. Patient Y - Overlooking Renal Impairment

A 60-year-old patient with a history of renal impairment presented with symptoms of a urinary tract infection (UTI). Initial urinalysis and symptoms were indicative of a bacterial UTI, leading to an antibiotic prescription.

While the diagnosis of a bacterial UTI was accurate, the healthcare provider failed to consider the patient's existing renal condition when prescribing Amoxicillin. The standard dose was prescribed, without any adjustments for renal function.

The patient took the antibiotic as prescribed but started to experience symptoms of toxicity, including severe nausea, vomiting, and confusion. Emergency hospitalization was required, where further tests revealed that the Amoxicillin levels in the bloodstream were dangerously high due to the patient's impaired kidney function.

This case serves as a cautionary tale about the importance of individualized treatment plans. Failure to adjust the antibiotic dose for renal function led to a life-threatening situation that could have been easily avoided with a more thorough patient evaluation.

These cautionary tales are intended to serve as educational narratives, emphasizing the need for proper diagnostic procedures, individualized treatment plans, and the responsible use of antibiotics like Amoxicillin. .

FAQS (FREQUENTLY ASKED QUESTIONS) ABOUT AMOXICILLIN

This chapter aims to address common questions and misconceptions, offering clear and comprehensive answers to help both patients and healthcare providers make informed decisions regarding antibiotic therapy.

Can Amoxicillin Treat Viral Infections?

One of the most common misconceptions about antibiotics, including Amoxicillin, is that they can treat viral infections like the common cold or the flu. This is incorrect. Antibiotics are specifically designed to target bacterial infections, not viruses. Using Amoxicillin for viral infections will not only be ineffective but will also contribute to antibiotic resistance. It's essential for healthcare providers to make a proper diagnosis before prescribing antibiotics and for patients to follow medical advice rather than self-medicating.

What Happens If I Miss a Dose?

Another frequent question revolves around missed doses. If you miss a dose of Amoxicillin, it's generally advised to take it as soon as you remember, unless it's almost time for your next dose. In that case, skip the missed dose and continue with your regular schedule. Do not double up on doses to make up for a missed one. Missing a dose can lead to suboptimal levels of the drug in your system, which can reduce its effectiveness and contribute to antibiotic resistance.

Can I Drink Alcohol While Taking Amoxicillin?

The interaction between alcohol and Amoxicillin is a common concern. While alcohol doesn't directly interfere with the effectiveness of Amoxicillin, it can have an additive effect on side effects like dizziness or upset stomach. Furthermore, excessive alcohol consumption can compromise your immune system, making it harder for your body to fight off infection. Therefore, it's generally advisable to limit alcohol intake while on Amoxicillin.

Is It Safe to Take Expired Amoxicillin?

The safety of using expired medications is a frequent query. While taking a dose or two of expired Amoxicillin is unlikely to cause harm, its effectiveness may be compromised. The drug may have degraded over time, reducing its potency. This can result in subtherapeutic levels in the blood, making it less effective in treating the infection and potentially contributing to antibiotic resistance.

Can Amoxicillin Affect Birth Control?

Many women are concerned about the interaction between antibiotics and oral contraceptives. Some antibiotics, including Amoxicillin, can potentially reduce the effectiveness of birth control pills. Although the evidence is not definitive, it's advisable to use an additional method of contraception while on antibiotics and for a short period afterward.

What Should I Do If I Experience Side Effects?

Experiencing side effects while on Amoxicillin is another frequent concern. Common side effects like mild nausea or diarrhea are usually not cause for alarm and may resolve on their own. However, symptoms like severe diarrhea, allergic reactions, or signs of anaphylaxis (like difficulty breathing) are medical emergencies that require immediate attention.

What Foods or Medications Should I Avoid?

Patients often wonder about food or drug interactions with Amoxicillin. While Amoxicillin is generally well-tolerated and has fewer interactions compared to some other antibiotics, it's crucial to discuss any over-the-counter medications, supplements, or herbal products you are taking with your healthcare provider.

Can Children Take Amoxicillin?

Amoxicillin is commonly prescribed for children to treat a variety of bacterial infections, including ear infections, strep throat, and pneumonia. Pediatric doses are usually calculated based on body weight and should be strictly followed. Parents and caregivers should administer the antibiotic as directed by the healthcare provider. Children may experience side effects like diarrhea, so monitoring for any adverse reactions is crucial. It is also essential to ensure that the child completes the entire course of the medication, even if they start to feel better, to prevent antibiotic resistance.

How Long Does It Take for Amoxicillin to Work?

Another common question is the time it takes for the antibiotic to start showing effects. Generally, patients may start to feel better within 24 to 48 hours of taking Amoxicillin. However, this does not mean the infection has been entirely eradicated. It's critical to complete the full course of the antibiotic as prescribed to ensure the bacteria are entirely eliminated, thus preventing a relapse or the development of antibiotic resistance.

Should I Take Amoxicillin with Food?

Amoxicillin can generally be taken with or without food. However, taking it with food may help reduce gastrointestinal side effects like nausea. Some formulations of Amoxicillin, such as extended-release tablets, may have specific instructions regarding food intake. Always follow the guidelines provided by your healthcare provider or pharmacist.

Can I Exercise While Taking Amoxicillin?

Physical activity and exercise are generally considered safe while taking Amoxicillin, unless you are experiencing symptoms like dizziness or lethargy, which could be side effects of the medication. It's advisable to monitor how your body responds to the antibiotic before engaging in strenuous exercise. If you experience any unusual symptoms, consult your healthcare provider.

Can Amoxicillin Treat Fungal Infections?

Amoxicillin is not effective against fungal infections like Candida. In fact, the use of antibiotics can sometimes lead to an overgrowth of fungus, resulting in conditions like oral thrush. If you suspect a fungal infection, consult your healthcare provider for appropriate antifungal treatment.

Is Amoxicillin Safe for Pets?

While Amoxicillin is sometimes prescribed for pets like dogs and cats, it should only be administered under veterinary supervision. The dosages for animals differ significantly from those for humans. Moreover, improper use of antibiotics in pets can also contribute to antibiotic resistance.

In summary, the FAQs section serves to clarify common misconceptions and provide valuable information to patients and healthcare providers alike. By addressing these additional questions, we aim to provide a comprehensive understanding of Amoxicillin usage, covering a range of scenarios and concerns that patients and healthcare providers may encounter.

Proper education and adherence to guidelines are essential steps in combating the increasing problem of antibiotic resistance and ensuring effective treatment. It's crucial for patients to consult their healthcare providers for any concerns or questions they may have regarding Amoxicillin use. Understanding the nuances of antibiotic therapy is not just the responsibility of healthcare providers but is a shared responsibility that includes patients.